PREGNANCY AND INFANTS:
MEDICAL, PSYCHOLOGICAL AND SOCIAL ISSUES

WORKING MEMORY IN INFANTS

PREGNANCY AND INFANTS: MEDICAL, PSYCHOLOGICAL AND SOCIAL ISSUES

Additional books in this series can be found on Nova's website under the Series tab.

Additional E-books in this series can be found on Nova's website under the E-book tab.

NEUROSCIENCE RESEARCH PROGRESS

Additional books in this series can be found on Nova's website under the Series tab.

Additional E-books in this series can be found on Nova's website under the E-book tab.

PREGNANCY AND INFANTS:
MEDICAL, PSYCHOLOGICAL AND SOCIAL ISSUES

WORKING MEMORY IN INFANTS

JING SUN

AND

NICHOLAS BUYS

Nova Biomedical Books

New York

For permission to use material from this book please contact us:
Telephone 631-231-7269; Fax 631-231-8175
Web Site: http://www.novapublishers.com

Library of Congress Cataloging-in-Publication Data

Working memory in infants / editors, Jing Sun and Nicholas Buys.
p. ; cm.
Includes bibliographical references and index.
ISBN 978-1-61122-742-0 (softcover)
1. Memory in infants. 2. Premature infants. I. Sun, Jing, Dr. II. Buys, Nicholas.
[DNLM: 1. Memory, Short-Term--physiology. 2. Frontal Lobe--growth & development. 3. Infant, Newborn--physiology. 4. Infant. 5. Memory Disorders. BF 378.S54] BF720.M45W67 2010 155.42'2312--dc22 2010041611

Published by Nova Science Publishers, Inc. † New York

Contents

Preface

Introduction: This study investigated working memory in preterm and full-term infants at 8 months after expected date of delivery. Working memory is defined as "the ability to maintain an appropriate problem solving set for the attainment of a future goal" (Welsh & Pennington, 1988, p. 201). An important characteristic of working memory is that it is prospective, that is, its purpose is to attain a goal, and it not only enables information to be held in mind but also to be manipulated. Working memory emerges in infancy and continues to develop throughout childhood. Working memory is believed to underlie some learning problems in children at school age. Although numerous studies have reported that the overall development of preterm infants is comparable to that of full-term infants at the same corrected age, it is unclear to what extent the development of specific cognitive abilities is affected by prematurity and/or other factors such as medical complications. As preterm infants have a high rate of learning difficulties, it is possible that factors associated with prematurity specifically affect the development of some regions of the brain associated with the regulation of working memory.

Methods: The current study aimed to examine the effects of maturation and length of exposure to extrauterine environmental stimuli on the development of working memory, by comparing the development of preterm infants with that of full-term infants at both the same corrected age and the same chronological age. A case-control study design was used for the study. Thirty-seven preterm infants without identified disabilities and 74 full-term and gender matched healthy full-term infants participated in the study. The preterm infants were all less than 32 weeks gestation and less than 1500 grams birthweight. All infants were assessed on working memory tasks at 8 months after the expected date of delivery (when preterm infants were actually 10-11 months chronological age).

Results: The findings of the study showed that preterm infants performed significantly more poorly than full-term infants at 8 months after the expected date of delivery on measures of working memory. The results suggest that the effects of maturation are greater than the effects of exposure to extrauterine environmental stimuli on the development of working memory. Furthermore, the preterm infants were divided into two subgroups on the basis of (a) low or high medical risk factors, (b) birthweight of < 1000 g versus 1000-1500 g, and (c) gestation age of < 28 weeks versus 28-32 weeks, in order to assess the effects of these variables on the performance of working memory. Medical risk, lower birthweight and lower gestation age were all found to adversely affect performance on working memory.

Discussions and conclusions: It is argued that medical risk, lower birthweight and lower gestation factors may influence the development of specific areas of the brain which govern working memory, and given that the prefrontal regions are particularly immature they may be especially vulnerable to damage or disruption. The present study provides further insights into the emergence of working memory in infants and the feasibility of evaluating these abilities in infants who are at risk for further learning difficulties and attention deficits.

Chapter I

Introduction

Advances in medical technology continue to improve the survival rate of preterm infants, so that increasing numbers of children who weigh < 1000 g at birth are surviving and entering the school system (Hack, Friedman, & Fanaroff, 1996; O'Shea, Klinepeter, Goldstein, Jackson, & Dillard, 1997). These at-risk children have been the focus of much research and many follow-up studies have identified a strong relationship between birthweight and learning development at school age (Rickards, Kelly, Doyle, & Callanan, 2001; Sostek, 1992; Taylor, Hack, Klein, & Schatschneider, 1995). Confounding this relationship, however, is the fact that as birthweight declines, the number and severity of perinatal complications experienced by infants is likely to increase (Klebanov, Brooks-Gunn, & McCormick, 1994).

Extensive attempts have been made to identify sensitive predictors of later learning problems in both term and preterm children (Aylward, 1994; G. Ross, Lipper, & Auld, 1996; Siegel, 1992). It has been accepted that learning problems have multiple determinants, and it is important to consider the interactions of biological factors (such as medical complications and genetic endowment), environmental factors (such as demographic factors, quality of educational experience, socioeconomic, and psychosocial factors), and developmental factors (such as specific cognitive abilities and general development as measured by infant general development assessment) (Koller, Lawson, Rose, Wallace, & McCarton, 1997; Laucht, Esser, & Schmidt, 1997). Frequently there is an association between perinatal risk and poor social circumstances. Several studies have demonstrated that social factors, particularly low educational level of the parents and socioeconomic status, play an important role in the intellectual outcome of both healthy full-term and preterm infants and those who had perinatal medical complications

(Landry, Denson, & Swank, 1997; Laucht et al., 1997; E. Roberts, Bornstein, Slater, & Barrett, 1999; Thompson et al., 1997).

The population of Very Low Birthweight (VLBW, birthweight between 1001-1500 grams) and Extremely Low Brithweight (ELBW, birthweight less than 1000 grams or 750 grams) infants is known to be at increased risk for a broad spectrum of health and developmental problems, and also an increased incidence of psychosocial disadvantages (e.g., poverty, single parenthood, youthful maternal age, and limited parental education), producing a "doubly vulnerable" population, which places their development in even greater jeopardy (Aylward, 1993, 1997). The assessment of subtle developmental and behavioural delays in infants is complicated, and currently there are few sensitive measures available for the early identification of learning problems in infants. Conventional developmental assessment tools, such as the Bayley Scales of Infant Development, (Bayley, 1993) only provide global indicators of development and fail to measure specific skills that may provide sensitive predictions of later learning.

The assessment of specific cognitive skills, in particular working memory, rather than a global development score in infancy, has been advocated by a number of investigators (Aylward, Pfeiffer, Wright, & Verhulst, 1989; McCall, 1994; Siegel, 1989). Working memory is defined as "the ability to maintain an appropriate problem solving set for the attainment of a future goal" (Welsh & Pennington, 1988, p. 201). Working memory deficits have been linked to a range of developmental problems, including attentional deficit disorder (ADD), learning difficulties, and autism, all of which are more prevalent in children born preterm (Gathercole & Pickering, 2000; Luciana, Lindeke, Georgieff, Mills, & Nelson, 1999). Studying a group of infants at high-risk for learning difficulties should make it easier to identify factors that are predictive of later learning problems. This may lead to a greater understanding of the etiology of these problems in all children.

In Welsh and Pennington's model of working memory, certain information remains at the forefront of cognition, despite distraction, and hence is active for the purpose of guiding appropriate responses. An important characteristic of working memory is that it is prospective, that is, its purpose is to attain a goal. Fuster (1997) suggested that this is achieved not only by holding information in mind, but also by guiding goal directed actions. Graham and Harris (1996) stated that working memory is also necessary in tasks which require strategy selection, monitoring, and revision of actions. This implies that working memory not only enables information to be held in mind but also to be manipulated. It is generally agreed that these behaviours are governed by the prefrontal cortex of the brain (Fuster,

1997; Goldman-Rakic, 1994). This part of the brain is late in developing and therefore may be particularly vulnerable to damage in preterm infants.

Evidence from Animal and Lesions Studies in Humans

Evidence for the link between working memory and prefrontal lobe has come from a wide range of sources including studies of the effects of brain lesions (Eslinger, Grattan, Damasio, & Damasio, 1992; Hecaen, 1964; Milner, 1963; Shallice & Burgess, 1991), neurophysiological, and neuroimaging investigations of animals, and both normal and clinical human populations (Grady, 1999; Hoon & Melhem, 2000; Jagust, 1999; Lepage et al., 1999; Marenco, Coppola, Daniel, Zigun, & Weinberger, 1993). Several researchers (i.e., Barkley, 1997; Fuster, 1997; Kaufer & Lewis, 1999) suggested that the frontal lobe may be divided into three regions: dorsolateral, orbital, and medial cortex. It has been shown that the dorsolateral region of the prefrontal cortex mediates the functioning of working memory (Fuster, 1997).

Originally, most experimental studies examining working memory consequences of damage to the dosolateral region of the prefrontal lobe was conducted on animals (Goldman-Rakic & Rosvold, 1972; Petrides, 1994, 1996). These studies, which involved ablation or temporary inactivation of the dorsolateral part of the prefrontal lobe of the brain, provided vital information about the location of various cognitive functions within the brain. In ablation studies, large lesions of the prefrontal cortex produced decrements in performance on the Delayed Response (DR) task which was designed to measure working memory in the literature (Diamond, 1985; Diamond & Doar, 1989). In the DR task, an infant sits before two identical hiding locations (e.g., cloth covers, cups or wells) that are separated by a small distance. While the infant watches, a desired object is hidden in one location, location A. After a delay, the infant is allowed to reach and search for the object. Then while the infant watches, the object is hidden at the second location, location B. After a delay, the infant is allowed to reach and search for the object. The sequence of hiding locations in A and B in the DR task is random. Temporary, reversible depression or inactivation of the cortex by cooling (Fuster, 1991), or the injection of drugs (Sawaguchi & Goldman-Rakic, 1994), induced a similar marked deterioration in performance on such tasks. The importance of these latter studies is that they showed that the effect was reversible and could be repeated on the same subject, clearly demonstrating that it was due to inactivity of the prefrontal cortex and not to some side effects of surgical intervention, and that it was consistent and repeatable. No deficits in DR task performance appeared on depressing or cooling other areas of the brain such as the parietal cortex. Although most of the above studies were conducted on adult primates, these studies provided vital information about a link between the prefrontal cortex and working memory.

Data on the effects of brain lesions on behaviour in humans are derived mainly from case reports of individuals who have sustained specific brain lesions (e.g., Guitton, Buchtel, & Douglas, 1985; Levine, 1993; Milner, 1963; Teuber & Rudel, 1962), or from studies of clinical populations who have sustained somewhat diffuse brain injuries (e.g., Benton, 1991; Levin, Song, Ewing-Cobbs, & Roberson, 2001; Mateer & Williams, 1991; McDowell, Whyte, & D'Esposito, 1997). Many of the findings from these clinical observations have now been corroborated and extended in normal subjects using neuroimaging techniques, such as magnetic resonance imaging (MRI), positron emission tomography (PET), and single photon emission computed tomography (e.g., Grady, 1999; Hoon & Melhem, 2000; Jagust, 1999). The evidence obtained suggests that damage to any part of the dorsolateral frontal lobe due to trauma, tumour, vascular accident or other disease processes produces deficits in working memory, leading to poor temporal integration of behaviour (Bohm, Katz-Salamon, Smedler, Lagercrantz, & Forssberg, 2002; Chui & Willis, 1999; Levin et al., 2001; Nakawatase, 1999; Rieger & Gauggel, 2002; Vasterling et al., 2002). The subject fails to remember information or is not motivated to remember, and has a limited capacity to adapt to new situations because of difficulties in planning future actions that deviate from ordinary routines.

Impairment of Working Memory

Patients with frontal lobe damage have consistently been found to display deficits in working memory on a large variety of different assessment tools. For example, a number of studies using DR tasks with visual, auditory, and kinesthetic stimuli have clearly demonstrated the difficulties experienced by patients with frontal lobe damage (Lewinsohn, Zieler, Libet, Eyeberg, & Nielson, 1972; Milner, 1968; Petrides, 1985; Stuss,

1991). For example, they could not do these tasks when time delays imposed by a research on a task. These problems with working memory are not seen in normal subjects and patients with other cortical lesions, such as temporal-lobe damage and posterior cortical lesions (Lewinsohn et al., 1972; Petrides, 1994).

The Development of Frontal Lobe in Human Infants

The prefrontal cortex is one of the last regions of the central nervous system to undergo full myelination, and developmental changes originating from frontal lobe development are evident in several periods of life (Thatcher, 1991). The most active periods of development of the prefrontal cortex appear to be in the first 2 years of life, then between 7 and 9 years, and finally in adolescence. The development of the frontal lobe in infants deserves particular mention because during this period remarkable and rapid changes occur in both the neural physiology and the behaviour of the human being. For the frontal cortex, the period of maximum synaptic excess appears to be in the second half of the first year (Huttenlocher, 1994), after which there occurs a protracted period of decline in synaptic density through selective elimination of little used pathways. Recent studies of human brain activity using positron emission tomography (PET) technique documented developmental changes in rates of glucose metabolism (Chugani & Phelps, 1990). These changes are characterised by a rise in metabolism in the frontal region at approximately 6-8 months of age, followed by a prolonged period of decline in rates of metabolism which parallels the decline in synaptic density (Chugani & Phelps, 1990). Thus, it seems that the significant and rapid changes related to anatomy and function of the fontal lobe occur in the second half of the first year after birth and continue more slowly after this early period.

There is ample evidence that working memory also develops dramatically during the second half of the first year of life. For example, infants can hold information in mind for increasing periods of time and use this information to direct and regulate their responses. Behaviours of this type have been shown in numerous studies to be related to the prefrontal cortex.

Bell and Fox (1992) further demonstrated a relationship between working memory and prefrontal lobe functioning and showed individual differences in frontal-brain electrical activity, as shown in EEG recordings and performance on the A*B* task. Infants at eight months of age who succeeded on the A*B* task exhibited greater power values in the frontal EEG during baseline recordings than infants who were unable to do the task (Bell, 1998; Bell & Fox, 1992).

Additional evidence for the importance of prefrontal cortex maturation for the development of working memory abilities has come from studies of children with phenylketonuria (A. Diamond, Prevor, Callender, & Druin, 1997). Even when treated, this genetically transmitted error of metabolism can have the specific consequence of reducing the levels of the neurotransmitter dopamine in the dorsolateral prefrontal cortex. This results in impaired performance on tasks thought to measure working memory, such as the A*B* task (Diamond, 1985; Diamond & Doar, 1989). The standard A*B* task was originally described by Piaget (1954) to measure the changes in the concept of object permanence in human infants. In Piaget's A*B* task, an infant sits before two identical hiding places, often referred to as occluders (e.g., two identical cloth covers or two identical lids) that are separated by a small distance. While the infant watches, a desired object is hidden in one location (A). After a delay, the infant is allowed to reach and search for the object. This hiding and search at location A is repeated. Then while the infant watches, the object is hidden at the second location (B). After the delay, the infant is allowed to reach and search for the object. Infants frequently make the error of searching again at location A, committing what is known as the classic A*B* error. Thus both electrophysiological and behavioural data provide support for the relation between the development of the prefrontal cortex and the emergence of working memory in the first year of life.

During this important maturation process in the first year of life, any damage or disturbance to the development of the prefrontal cortex due to disease, trauma, or conditions associated with perinatal risk factors (i.e., medical complications, extremely low birthweight, shorter gestation age) may therefore lead to working memory dysfunctioning. Diamond and Goldman-Rakic (1986) used animal models to examine whether lesions of the dorsolateral prefrontal cortex would have the same effect on infant monkeys as on adult monkeys. Two of the infant rhesus monkeys were tested longitudinally on the A*B* and the DR tasks. They received bilateral lesions of the dorsolateral prefrontal cortex at 5½ months. They were then tested on the A*B* task at 6 months. The findings showed that the infant monkeys that had the prefrontal lesions displayed poorer performance on the A*B* task than their age mates who did not have the prefrontal lesions. The lesions produced the same effect in infant monkeys as they did in adult monkeys with prefrontal lesions: they all reached incorrectly when the delay increased to 2-5 seconds s after the toy changed to the new hiding position.

Damage to the prefrontal lobe due to trauma and disease in infancy may have lifelong effects on working memory abilities, and may cause learning difficulties during school years (Eslinger et al., 1992; Scheibel & Levin, 1997). In comparison with adults, childhood frontal lobe lesions produce a more pervasive impairment, interfering with the acquisition of age-appropriate working memory skills. Most studies on the relationship between working memory development and frontal lobe damage in children are based on older children (Eslinger, Biddle, Pennington, & Page, 1999; Mateer & Williams, 1991). However, a recent case study by Anderson, Damasio, Tranel, and Damasio (2000) reported that an infant who had right frontal region damage at 3 months showed severe learning difficulties and behavioural problems at school, and failure in career development in adulthood despite average intelligence (as measured by traditional intelligence tests at school age and during adulthood). The study found that the impairments largely reflected a failure to develop working memory. These findings are consistent with the notion that early damage to prefrontal regions can lead to severe disruption of working memory, while not significantly affecting many aspects tapped by standard intelligence tests. They also suggest that the prefrontal cortex may have limited neuronal plasticity which contributes to poor working memory if the damage occurs early. This may be due to disruption to the laying down of the neural architectures which are viewed as the foundation of cognitive development. A detailed examination of the relationship between prefrontal cortex development and the development of working memory in a large sample of human infants has not been possible because of the relative lack of obvious prefrontal lesions in infants and the expense and lack of availability of neural imaging technology.

The prefrontal cortex of infants who are born preterm is even more immature and prone to damage from the multitude of adverse medical complications to which these frail infants may be exposed. Lesions or atypical development of the prefrontal cortex occurring as a consequence of these hazardous events may have a detrimental effect on the development of working memory which may have long-term consequences in terms of learning difficulties at school age. Indeed it has been found that children born preterm are at an increased risk for learning difficulties and attentional deficits when they reach school age and it has been suggested that this may be due to early abnormality in the development of the prefrontal cortex and consequently of working memory (Harvey, O'Callaghan, & Mohay, 1999; Luciana et al., 1999).

Failure of working memory has been shown to underlie learning difficulties and attention deficits in children and these problems are particularly common in children born preterm. Historically, the assessment of working memory in infants was thought impossible. However, recent neuropsychological research has suggested that the A*B* task provide avenues for research on working memory.

This study was undertaken to compare the performance of preterm and full-term infants of the same corrected age (8 months) age and 10-11 month chronological age on tests related to working memory.

The following two hypotheses will be tested through the study:

Hypothesis 1: There will be significant difference between preterm and full-term infants of the same chronological age in the performance of working memory task (i.e., exposure to extrauterine environmental stimuli is the key factor influencing the development of working memory.

Hypothesis 2: There will be significant difference between preterm and full-term infants of the same corrected age in the performance of working memory task (i.e., maturation of the central nervous system from the time of conception is the key factors influencing the development of working memory).

Chapter II

Methods

Study Design

This research involves the comparison of a cohort of ELBW infants (n = 37) and two comparison groups of full-term infants (n = 37 in each group) matched for gender and the age since expected date of delivery. The purpose of having two full-term comparison groups is to increase the statistical power. All infants were assessed on the working memory task. This measure formed the dependent variable.

Infants were also assessed on the confounding factors in the present study: perinatal variables which consist of medical complications, birthweight, and gestation age. All infants were assessed on the above variables at 8 months after the expected date of delivery (preterm infants were 10 to 11 months chronological age at this time). Term infants were reassessed at an age equivalent to the chronological age of the matched preterm infant at the time of the first assessment. This retest provided a comparison with the preterm infants on the basis of chronological age.

Participants

Participants consisted of two groups – preterm and fullterm infants.

1. Preterm infants: The mothers of 41 preterm infants, who attended the Growth and Development Unit at Mater Children's Hospital in Brisbane, Australia, responded to an invitation to participate in this study. These preterm infants were all born at the Mater Mothers' Hospital, Brisbane,

Australia, between May 1998 and July 1999. Inclusion criteria for preterm infants were:

- < 1500 g birthweight,
- < 32 weeks of gestation,
- eight months of age after expected date of delivery,
- no evidence of severe visual, auditory or neurological impairment, or severe congenital anomalies,
- living in the Brisbane metropolitan area, and
- mother was English-speaking.

Of the 41 preterm infants, 37 were included in the study group. Two infants were excluded from the study due to severe intellectual and neurological problems and two other infants were excluded from the data analysis due to errors in the administration of some of the test items. There were two sets of twins and one set of triplets.

2. Full-term Infants: Names and addresses of potential full-term comparison infants who were the same sex as the matched preterm infants, born at the Mater Mothers' Hospital on the same expected date of delivery, were obtained from medical records at the hospital. Parents were then contacted by a letter, and provided with an information sheet, and a follow-up telephone call. A total of 207 letters were sent, and of these 74 mothers of infants with birth weights of > 2500g were selected to match the corresponding preterm infants on a first-come basis. Inclusion criteria for full-term infants were:

- > 2500 grams birthweight,
- 38-42 weeks of gestation,
- same sex as matched preterm infant,
- born on the same expected date of delivery as the matched preterm infant,
- no evidence of perinatal complications or congenital abnormalities,
- living in the Brisbane metropolitan area,
- mother was English speaking, and
- developmentally normal

In summary, all infants recruited into this study were born at the same hospital and tested at eight months (+ or - 2 weeks) after the expected date of delivery. Full term infants were reassessed when they were 10-11 month chronological age. All subjects lived within a 50-kilometre radius of the Mater Mothers' Hospital and did not have identifiable disabilities at the time of assessment.

Participation in the project was voluntary and informed consent was obtained from at least one parent of each child. Ethical approval for the project was obtained from the Mater Children's and Mater Mothers' Hospital Ethics Committees, and the Queensland University of Technology Research Ethics Committee.

Working Memory Task

The assessment of working memory was based on a task derived from the A*B* and DR tasks which have been described in the literature (Diamond, 1985; Diamond & Doar, 1989). In the A*B* task, an infant sits before two identical hiding locations (e.g., cloth covers, cups or wells) that are separated by a small distance. While the infant watches, a desired object is hidden in one location, location A. After a delay, the infant is allowed to reach and search for the object. This hiding and searching at location A is repeated. Then while the infant watches, the object is hidden at the second location, location B. After a delay, the infant is allowed to reach and search for the object. Infants frequently make the error of searching again at location A committing what is known as the classic A*B* error. The sequence of hiding locations in the DR task is random, whereas the hiding locations in the A*B* task are determined by the number of correct searches at location A.

Procedure

The administration procedure is described below.

1) *Materials.* The following materials were used for the Infant Working Memory task: one yellow cup (used to cover the toys), two red cups, three blue cups, and three small toys for hiding under the cups.
2) *Pre-test.* This involved the experimenter putting a toy on the table in front of the infant while the infant was watching. The infants were allowed to retrieve the toy immediately to test whether they could reach it. If it was unclear whether the infant had reached for

the toy (e.g., if the infant showed an interest in the examiner or waited for several seconds before reaching to the toy), this procedure was repeated.

Ability to successfully retrieve the hidden objects is influenced by the infant's interest in and attention to the task (Horobin & Acredolo, 1986). To maintain infant's attention to the task, the colours of the occluders (the cups under which the goal objects were hidden), were changed at set points in the test administration.

Administration of the Infant Working Memory Task

1-cup task. The Infant Working Memory task started with a 1-cup task. One yellow opaque cup and three small round toys were used. A toy was placed directly in front of the infant, at a distance of approximately 20 cm. While the child watched, the opaque yellow cup was placed by the examiner over the toy so that the toy was invisible. For this trial and all subsequent trials the mother was asked to prevent the infant from reaching by gently holding him/her whilst the object was being covered and also during the imposition of a delay between hiding and retrieving the object. She was instructed, prior to the task, to release her child when the examiner said "find the toy." The infant's ability to remove the occluder and reach for the object underneath was then noted. Three trials were given for each of the delay periods (0, 4 and 10 seconds).

2-cup task. For the 2-cup task, two red opaque cups and the same three toys were used. One cup was positioned 11 cm to the right of the infant's midline, at a distance of 20 cm from the infant. The other was positioned 11 cm to the left, also at a distance of 20 cm from the infant. Testing began by positioning the goal object in front of the cup on the infant's left hand side. The cup was then moved to cover the object. The infant was then permitted to retrieve the object and allowed a few seconds to play with it. The toy was hidden in the following positions: right, right, left, left, and right for the remaining 5 trials. Then the delay time between hiding the object and retrieving was increased to 2 seconds. For the 2 seconds delayed period trial, the order for hiding the toy was: right, left, left, right, right, and left. The hiding locations for the 4 s delay was the same as that of the 0 s delay and the hiding locations for the 10 s delay was the same as for the 2 seconds delayed time condition.

3-cup task. In the 3-cup task, three blue cups and the same toys were used. In this condition, the toy was always hidden to the left and the right side of the infant and never in the middle. The order for the hiding location was the same as for the 2-cup condition. For the 2- and 3-cup difficulty level, the toy was always hidden on the left side first, because perseverative reaching has been demonstrated to be more common on an infant's right side (Hofstadter & Reznick, 1996).

For the 1-cup task, three trials were presented at each time delay of the task. From the 2-cup to 3-cup Infant Working Memory task, six trials were presented at each time delay of the task. Three round toys with three colours (red, yellow, and blue) were used as objects for hiding under the cups. These three toys were used for each trial each for the first three trials at each time delay level based on the colour sequence of red, yellow, and blue. The procedure for the presentation of toys were the same for the second three trials at each time delay level. During the inter-trial (i.e., between infant's retrieval and the preparation of next trial) interval, the experimenter gave the hidden toy to the infant to play with for approximately 20 s while the next trial was prepared. The inter-trial interval was about 20 seconds. A summary of the tasks is presented in Table 1.

Table 1. ***Infant Working Memory Task***

Tasks	Number of hiding places	Occluder (cup/s)	Delay time between hiding and reaching	Location of hidden object
1 cup	1	Yellow cup	Level 1: 0 s delay Level 2: 4 s delay Level 3: 10 s delay	
2 cups	2	Red Cups	Level 1: 0 s delay Level 2: 2 s delay Level 3: 4 s delay Level 4: 10 s delay	L **R** R **L** L **R** R **L** L **R** R **L** L **R** R **L** L **R** R **L** L **R** R **L**
3 cups	3	Blue cups	Level 1: 0 s delay Level 2: 2 s delay Level 3: 4 s delay Level 4: 10 s delay	L **R** R **L** L **R** R **L** L **R** R **L** L **R** R **L** L **R** R **L** L **R** R **L**

Note. R in the table refers to the right side, L refers to the left side of the infant. The bold type refers to the change to a new hiding position that provided a measure of inhibition to a prepotent response.

Criteria Used for Termination and Continuation of the Task

Each infant was tested on the 1-cup, 2-cup, and 3-cup tasks. In each of these conditions, the infant started from the easiest level of time delay, 0 seconds. If the infant failed to reach to the appropriate occluder on three consecutive trials at any delay level, the next trial was administered with one extra cup and 0 s delay, otherwise testing continued at the next level of delay with the same number of cups. The criteria used for terminating the task or moving to the next level are described in more detail below.

1) 1-cup task. Three presentations of this task could be given at each time delay (0, 4, 10 s). If the infant succeeded in removing the cup and obtaining the object underneath within the time limit on at least two of three presentations, then the task was administered at next level of time delay. If the infant failed to obtain the object on all three trials at a given time delay, following completion of three trials at 10 s delay the examiner moved on to the 2-cup task with a 0 s time delay.
2) 2-cup task. Six presentations of the 2-cup task were given at each delay time. There were four delay times (0, 2, 4, and 10 s), making a total of 24 trials. If the infant succeeded in reaching to the correct position on at least three consecutive trials on a given time delay, the next level of time delay was then presented. During the 2-cup task, if the infant failed to reach to the appropriate occluder on three consecutive trials at any delay level, testing of the 2-cup task was terminated, and the 3-cup task was administered with 0 s time delay.
3) 3-cup task. The criterion to pass this task was the same as in the 2-cup task. In this condition, if the infant failed to retrieve the toy on three consecutive trials at any delay level, the tester stopped the testing.

Scoring Scheme for Working Memory

As shown in Table 1, finding a hidden object in the 1-cup task requires infants to remember the hidden object rather than a location, and to be able to reach the hidden object. These are the criteria for the infants to perform the Infant Working Memory task. Finding a hidden object in location A in the 2- and 3-cup tasks requires working memory for location. Increasing the delay time between hiding and retrieval increases the difficulty of the task for infants (Diamond, 1993).

Therefore working memory was scored on the memory for location, and this was scored on the basis of the 2- and 3-cup tasks in location A. A score of one was awarded if the infant remembered the location of the toy on the first trial of both 2- and 3-cup tasks, and on subsequent trials when the hiding position was the same position as on the previous trial (i.e., all the A trials which are the ones not in bold type in Table 1). The task administration was organised so that this was always the 1st, 3rd and 5th trial at each time delay level. The total number of correct trials from all A trials attempted was then calculated. Possible scores ranged from 0-12 for both the 2- and 3-cup tasks (i.e., a possible overall total range of 0-24).

Data Analysis

All data were analysed using the SPSS package version 17.0. Each preterm infant had two comparison term infants matched for gender and age. The comparison between the study group and comparison groups on working memory tasks at eight months corrected age and 10-11 months chronological age was analysed by multivariate analysis of variance to test Hypothesis 1 and Hypothesis 2.

If there was a significant difference between preterm and full-term infants, the confounding variables which may explain this difference were examined. Perinatal variables which might confound the effects of prematurity, such as medical risks, birthweight, and gestation age, were also examined using ANOVA to compare the differences between the two preterm and one full-term infant groups.

Chapter III

Results

The aim of this analysis was to compare the performance of preterm and full-term infants of the same chronological age (i.e., 10-11 months after expected date of delivery) and the same corrected age (i.e., eight months after expected date of delivery) on working memory task.

Table 2. Comparison of Preterm and Full-term Infants on working memory Tasks at 10-11 Month Chronological Age and Eight Months Corrected Age

Executive function	Preterm	Full-term group	F	p
1.Working memory M (SD) Chronological age	 5.75 (3.11) 1.67 (.57) A1	 13.42(4.01) 2.50 (.40) A2	 21.78	 .00
2. Working memory M (SD) Corrected age	 5.75 (3.11) A1	 9.40 (4.45) A2	 11.82	 .00

The univariate ANOVAs showed that each of the components of working memory contributed significantly to the differences between groups for working memory measure. There was a significant difference between the preterm group and full-term infants group on the working memory task.

There were significant differences between preterm and full-term infants at 10-11 months chronological age in the performance of working memory. Preterm infants showed significantly poorer performance than the full-term infant groups on working memory. These results supported Hypothesis 1, which stipulated that there will be significant difference between preterm and full-term infants of the same chronological age in the performance of working memory task (i.e., exposure to extrauterine environmental stimuli is the key factor influencing the development of working memory

It was also found that there were significant differences between preterm and full-term infant groups at eight months corrected age on working memory. Specifically, preterm infants as a group had significantly poorer performances on working memory compared with the full-term infant groups at eight months corrected age. These results supported Hypothesis 2, that postulated that the performance of preterm infants is different to full-term infants of the same corrected age on measure of working memory.

From this point, all of the analyses refer to the performance of infants at 8 months corrected age, and aim to identify those factors which might contribute to the differences in performance on working memory task between preterm and term infants.

It is possible that some factors associated with being preterm affected performance of working memory more than prematurity per se. These factors include medical complications, lower birthweight and shorter gestation age. Further analyses were conducted to assess the effect of perinatal variables which might have significantly affected preterm infants' performance on the working memory measures.

Preterm infants were firstly grouped on the basis of their severity of medical complication as follows. None of the full term infants had serious perinatal complications and they were combined to form one group.

1) high-risk preterm group (n = 18), group 1;
2) low-risk preterm group (n = 19), group 2; and,
3) no medical complications (term infants n = 74), group 3.

The results of high risk preterm infants, low-risk preterm infants and full term infants are shown in Table 3.

The preterm infants who had a high medical risk in the perinatal period performed worse than those who did not have these medical risk factors on working memory, although the differences in performance were not statistically significant. The scores of both the preterm infant groups were lower than those of full-term infants on working memory measure. These differences reached statistical significance between both groups of preterm infants and full-term infants on working memory. The difference between preterm infants who had high medical risk and full-term infants was greater than that between low-risk infants and full-term infants on working memory, suggesting that medical risk influences the development of working memory.

Table 3. The Comparison of Preterm Infants at High Medical Risk, Low Medical Risk, and Full-term Infants on Measures of Executive Function and Sustained Attention at Eight Months Corrected Age

Variables	High-risk preterm infants	Low-risk preterm infants	Full-term Infants	*F*	*p*	Tukey's HSD
Working memory *M (SD)*	4.61 (2.95)**A1**	6.84 (2.93) **A2**	9.36 (4.22) **A3**	12.34	.00	A1 vs.A3 (.00) A2 vs.A3 (.03)

Preterm infants were grouped on the basis of their birthweights as follows. None of the full-term infants was low birthweight and they were combined to form one group:

1) < 1000 g birthweight ($n = 21$), group 1;
2) 1000-1500 g birthweight group ($n = 16$), group 2; and,
3) normal birthweight group (term infants, $n = 74$), group 3.

The results of infants with less than 1000g birthweight, infants with 1001-1500g birthweight and normal birthweight infants are shown in Table 4.

Table 4. The Comparison of < 1000 g Birthweight Infants, 1000-1500 g Birthweight Infants and Full-term Infants on Working Memory Mmeasure at Eight Months Corrected Age

Variab-les	< 1000 g birthweight	1000-1500 g birthweight	Full-term Infants	*F*	*p*	Tukey's HSD
Working memory *M (SD)*	5.23 (3.36)**A1**	6.43(2.70) **A2**	9.36 (4.22)**A3**	11.01	.00	A1 vs.A3 (.00) A2 vs.A3 (.02)

The preterm infants who had < 1000 g birthweight performed worse than those who had ≥ 1000 g birthweight on working memory although the differences in performance were not statistically significant. The scores of both groups of preterm infants were poorer than those of full-term infants on working memory. These differences were statistically significant between both groups of preterm infants and full-term infants on working memory. Thus the differences between the preterm infants who had < 1000 g birthweight and full-term infants appear greater than that between the infants with ≥ 1000 g birthweight and full-term infants on working memory, suggesting that ELBW may significantly influence the development of working memory.

Preterm infants were grouped on the basis of their gestation age. None of the full-term infants had low gestation age and they were combined to form one group.

1) 28 weeks gestation age ($n = 15$), group 1;
2) 28 to 32 weeks gestation age ($n = 22$), group 2; and
3) normal gestation age (full-term infants, $n = 74$), group 3.

Table 5 shows that scores were poorer for the infants < 28 weeks gestation than for the preterm infants with ≥ 28 weeks gestation on working memory, and the scores of both groups of preterm infants were poorer than those of full-term infants on working memory. These differences reached statistical significance between preterm infants and the group of full-term infants on working memory.

Table 5. The Comparison of < 28 Weeks Gestation Infants, 28-32 Weeks Gestation Infants and Full-term Infants on Working Memory Measure at Eight Months Corrected Age

Variables	< 28 weeks *M (SD)*	28-32 weeks *M (SD)*	Full-term Infants *M (SD)*	*F*	*p*	Tukey's HSD
Working memory *M (SD)*	5.53 (2.66) **A1**	5.90 (3.43) **A2**	9.36 (4.22) **A3**	10.54	.00	A1 vs.A3 (.00) A2 vs.A3 (.00)

Chapter IV

Discussion

Preterm and full-term infants of the same chronological age and same corrected age were compared on measures of working memory in order to assess the differential effects of maturation (biological maturity) and length of exposure to extrauterine environmental stimuli on the development of these abilities. Although a number of studies suggest that global development seems to be largely the result of maturational influence (Hunt & Rhodes, 1977; Rutter, 1992; Ungerer & Sigman, 1983), others have reported that "neural sculpting" occurs as the result of exposure to environmental influences (Campos, Kermoian, Witherington, Chen, & Dong, 1997; Dawson et al., 1999). Currently little is known about the impact of the environment on the development of brain mechanisms that mediate specific cognitive abilities, such as working memory.

It was found that preterm infants were inferior to full-term infants on working memory tasks at both the same chronological age and the same corrected age, but the differences in performance were much less when the infants were compared at the same corrected age. This suggests that maturation had a greater impact than exposure to environmental stimuli on the development of working memory. However, as differences between the preterm and full term infants remained even when they were compared on corrected age, other factors must also have impact on the development of working memory in these infants. It was also found that high-risk perinatal complications, extremely low birthweight (<1000 g) and very low gestation age (< 28 weeks) were associated with poor performance on working memory task.

Preterm infants represent a heterogeneous population which varies with respect to gestation age, birthweight, adequacy of interuterine growth, and the diversity of medical complications to which they may have been exposed. All too often in the literature these differences have been ignored and data from preterm infants has been lumped together. It is however essential to consider the effect which these factors may have over and above the effects of prematurity per se.

The perinatal risk factors examined in the present study were high medical risk, extremely low birthweight, and shorter gestation age. A "high medical risk preterm infant" was defined as an infant who had one or more of the following perinatal medical complications, previously identified as associated with poor outcomes. (Cohen, Parmelee, Beckwith, & Sigman, 1986; Gregoire, Lefebvre, & Glorieux, 1998; Hertzig, 1981; Landry et al., 1997; Msall et al., 1991; Piecuch, Leonard, Cooper, & Sehring, 1997; Pine, Jackson, & Bennett, 1995; Smith et al., 1996; Sostek, 1992; van de Bor, den Ouden, & Guit, 1992). These were: Home Oxygen Dependency, Cerebral Ventricular Hemorrhage, Ventricular Dilatation, and Periventricular Hemorrhage-Intraventricular Hemorrhage. VD did not occur in any of the infants in the present study so it was not used for the analysis. Eighteen infants fell into this "high medical risk" category, and the remaining 19 preterm infants were defined as "low medical risk."

ELBW was defined as birthweight < 1000 g. Preterm infants in the < 1000 g birthweight group did not differ from the preterm infants with ≥ 1000 g birthweight group with regards to medical risk status. Two gestation age groups comprised infants with gestation age < 28 weeks and preterm infants with ≥ 28 weeks gestation age. Infants with gestation age < 28 weeks were regarded as having shorter gestation age. Likewise, preterm infants born at < 28 weeks gestation were not significantly different to those with 28-32 weeks gestation in terms of medical risk status. There was therefore an opportunity to consider the effect of birthweight and gestation age independent of medical complications.

In each case, the high-risk group (i.e., the medical complications group, the <1000 g birthweight group, and the < 28 weeks gestation group) performed more poorly than their low risk counterparts (i.e., the low medical risk group, the > 1000 g birthweight group, and the > 28 weeks gestation group) on working memory measure although these differences did not reach statistical significance. The performance of both the high risk and low risk preterm groups on measure of working memory were also consistently poorer than that of the full-term group, and this reached levels of statistical significance more frequently for the high risk preterm groups than for the low risk groups. The results of the effects of perinatal factors on the performance of working memory are summarised in Table 6 below. These findings suggest that medical risk, lower birthweight, and lower gestation age adversely affect performance on working memory measure.

Table 6. Influence of Perinatal Risk Factors on Performance of Working Memory Measure When Compared to Full-term Infants

Variables	Medical risk		Birthweight		Gestation age	
	High risk p	Low risk p	< 1000 g p	> 1000 g p	< 28 weeks p	> 28 weeks p
Working memory	.03*	.00***	.00***	.02*	.00***	.00***

Note. The figures in the table above are summarized from Tables 3, 4 and 5. Significant difference between preterm infant group and full-term infant group: *$p < .05$,
** $p < .01$, *** $p < .001$.

The findings of this study are consistent with those of other researchers, who have reported that perinatal risk factors influence cognitive development during the first year of life (Molfese & Thomson, 1985; Piper, Kunos, Willis, & Mazer, 1985; G. Ross, Tesman, Auld, & Nass, 1992). Similar deficits in working memory have also been reported in studies of school age children who were born preterm and who experienced high medical risk (Luciana et al., 1999; Taylor, Klein, Minich, & Hack, 2000). For example, Luciana et al. (1999) found that preterm born children at 7 to 9 years of age who had high medical risk differed from full-term infants on working memory tasks, and Taylor, Klein, et al. (1998) also suggested that medical risk may influence the long term developmental outcomes of preterm infants.

The results are also consistent with previous studies of children with extremely low birthweight, whether defined as birthweight < 1000 g (Harvey et al., 1999) or < 750 g (Taylor, Klein et al., 2000), which have reported lower scores on the performance of working memory tasks. However the children in these studies were older than the children in the present study. The effect of SGA may also influence the performance of working memory in the preterm infants with < 1000 g birthweight group in the current study. For example, the poorer performance of the ELBW infants on working memory may have been due to the fact that there were eight SGA infants in the ELBW group. Several studies, such as that of McCarton et al. (1996) have reported that SGA preterm infants tend to perform more poorly than their AGA counterparts on general developmental assessment measures. In the current study, SGA preterm infants tended to show poorer scores on the working memory measure than AGA preterm infants, but these differences did not reach statistically significant differences as the number of SGA infants in the present study was too small. Evidence for direct central nervous system effects of intrauterine undernutrition is primarily based on animal studies. Laboratory studies in rats and guinea pigs that have experienced intrauterine growth retardation have shown decreased brain weight, and reduced amount of brain DNA, protein, and myelin lipids (Neville & Chase, 1971). While extrapolation from animal studies is questionable this does raise the possibility that SGA infants may experience cognitive impairments as the result of reduced brain growth.

This study appears to be the first to examine the effect of gestation age on the performance of working memory. The effects of gestation age on subsequent cognitive development has been the topic of considerable debate. Many studies have included a heterogeneous group of preterm infants with a wide range of gestation ages. The effects of gestation age on subsequent development have consequently often been confounded by a higher incidence of perinatal complications and poor psychomotor development in the infants of lower gestation age (Duffy, Als, & McAnulty, 1990; Emsley, Wardle, Sims, Cheswick, & Souza, 1998; Eyal, 1993; Synnes et al., 1994; The Victorian Infant Collaborative Study Group, 1997). In this study, both preterm infants with < 28 weeks gestation and infants with 28-32 weeks gestation had lower scores than the full-term infants on working memory. The differences between both preterm groups and full-term infants reached statistical significance on measure of working memory. This suggests that a shorter gestation age is no more detrimental to performance in these areas than prematurity per se.

There is considerable evidence that tasks which require the holding of information in memory involve the dorsolateral prefrontal cortex (Diamond, Kirkham, & Amso, 2002; J. R. J. Roberts & Pennington, 1996). The deficits in working memory observed in the high perinatal risk groups may be associated with the adverse effects of these perinatal risk factors on the prefrontal cortex which is very immature and sensitive in the preterm infants (Aylward, 1993; Diamond & Lee, 2000; Fletcher et al., 1996). Mouradian, Als, and Coster (2000) suggested that deficits in working memory might be due to late maturing cortical organization, particularly of the prefrontal regions. Myelination of the brain has been demonstrated to occur in a systematic fashion starting at the end of the first trimester and continuing at least until the end of the second year (Battin et al., 1998). Between 23 and 32 weeks of gestation, structural differentiation of the central nervous system is at its most rapid (i.e., neuronal differentiation, glial cell growth, myelination, axonal and dendritic growth and synapse formation). The preterm infants in the present study were born between 24 to 32 weeks gestation just at this time of brain development. Most of these preterm infants were in the Neonatal Intensive-care Unit for up to three months after they were born. The environment in the Neonatal Intensive-care Unit may not be conductive to the development of the brain and the perinatal risk factors which occurred during this period may have further adversely affect brain development. The prefrontal cortex, which appears to play a central role in regulating working memory, is a late maturing area of the brain, and is consequently likely to be particularly vulnerable to damage in preterm infants (Gilles, Shankle, & Dooling, 1983). Those preterm infants with these detrimental perinatal events are at particular risk for the abnormal prefrontal cortex functioning, hence the deficits in working memory.

The deficits of working memory observed in preterm infants may have long term consequences in terms of learning difficulties at school age. During school years, children born preterm who experienced high perinatal risks (i.e., high medical risks, extremely low birthweight, shorter gestation age) during the perinatal period have been found to have higher rates of deficits in cognitive and neuropsychological abilities, mathematics achievement, and adaptive behaviours, as well as higher rates of special education placements as compared with their full-term counterparts (Hack et al., 1996; Luciana et al., 1999; Taylor, Anselmo, Foreman, Schatschneider, & Angelopoulos, 2000; Taylor et al., 1998). It is possible that this is due to early abnormality in the development of the prefrontal cortex and consequent working memory impairment. Anderson et al. (2000) suggested that this might possibly result in inability to ever acquire aspects of working memory.

In summary, there were significant differences between preterm and full-term infants' scores on working memory at both 10-11 month chronological age and eight month corrected age. Medical risk factors, extremely low birthweight, and shorter gestation age confounded the effects of prematurity for working memory.

Limitation of the Study

There are several limitations of this study. First, due to the restricted timeframe, long-term outcomes cannot be assessed. Hence a link cannot be made to the preterm infants between the deficits in working memory found in the present study and learning difficulties in school. Second, the examiner was not blind to the preterm/term status of the infants and this may have affected the administration and coding of the tests. Third, the relatively small sample of preterm infants who could be recruited within the time constraints for the present study restricted the range for statistical analyses that could be carried out and thus limited their power. Finally, the strict selection criteria chosen to yield a group of relatively healthy preterm infants may have biased the sample and made it unrepresentative of the general population of every preterm infant. For the above reasons the results should be interpreted with some caution.

Chapter V

Conclusion

Differences were found between preterm and full-term infants on measures of working memory at both the same corrected and same chronological age. Maturation was found to be an important factor influencing the development of working memory. However other factors associated with prematurity were also found to affect performance on working memory measure.

The present research examined the factors which may significantly affect the differences between preterm and full-term infants. In particular, high medical risk, lower birthweight, and shorter gestation age all affected the differences between preterm and full-term infants on of working memory measure.

References

Anderson, S. W., Damasio, H., Tranel, D., & Damasio, A. R. (2000). Long-term sequelae of prefrontal cortex damage acquired in early childhood. *Developmental Neuropsychology, 18*(3), 281-290.

Aylward, G. P. (1993). Perinatal asphyxia: Effects of biological and environmental risks. *Clinics in Perinatology, 20*, 433-449.

Aylward, G. P. (1994). Update on early developmental neuropsychological assessment: The early neuropsychological optimality rating scales. In M. G. Tramontana & S. R. Hooper (Eds.), *Advances in child neuropsychology* (pp. 172-200). New York: Springer-Verlag.

Aylward, G. P. (1997). *Infant and early childhood neuropsychology*. New York: Plenum Press.

Aylward, G. P., Pfeiffer, S. I., Wright, A., & Verhulst, S. J. (1989). Outcome studies of low birth weight infants published in the last decade: A meta-analysis. *Journal of Pediatrics, 115*, 515-520.

Barkley, R. A. (1997). Behavioral inhibition, sustained attention, and executive functions: Constructing a unifying theory of ADHD. *Psychological Bulletin, 121*(1), 65-94.

Battin, M. R., Maalouf, E. F., Counsell, S. J., Herlihy, A. H., Rutherford, M. A., Azzopardi, D., et al. (1998). Magnetic resonance imaging of the brain in very preterm infants: Visualization of the germinal matrix, early myelination, and cortical folding. *Pediatrics, 101*(6), 957-962.

Bayley, N. (1993). *Bayley scale of infant development: Manual* (2nd ed.). San Antonio, TX: The Psychological Corporation.

Bell, M. A. (1998). Frontal lobe function during infancy: Implications for the development of cognition and attention. In J. E. Richards (Ed.), *Cognitive neuroscience of attention: A developmental perspective* (pp. 287-316). Mahwah, NJ: Lawrence Erlbaum.

Bell, M. A., & Fox, N. A. (1992). The relations between frontal brain electrical activity and cognitive development during infancy. *Child Development, 63*, 1142-1163.

Benton, A. (1991). Prefrontal injury and behavior in children. *Developmental Neuropsychology, 7*(3), 275-281.

Bohm, B., Katz-Salamon, M., Smedler, A., Lagercrantz, H., & Forssberg, H. (2002). Developmental risks and protective factors for influencing cognitive outcome at 5 1/2 years of age in very-low-birthweight children. *Developmental Medicine and Child Neurology, 44*, 508-516.

Campos, J. J., Kermoian, R., Witherington, D., Chen, H., & Dong, Q. (1997). Activity, attention and developmental transitions in infancy. In P. J. Lang & R. F. Simons (Eds.), *Attention and orienting: Sensory and motivational processes* (pp. 393-415). Mahwah, NJ: Lawrence Erlbaum.

Chugani, H. T., & Phelps, M. E. (1990). Imaging human brain development with positron emission tomography. *Journal of Nuclear Medicine, 32*, 23-25.

Chui, H., & Willis, L. (1999). Vascular diseases of the frontal lobes. In B. L. Miller & J. L. Cummings (Eds.), *The human frontal lobes: Functions and disorders* (pp. 370-402). New York: The Guilford Press.

Cohen, S. E., Parmelee, A. H., Beckwith, L., & Sigman, M. (1986). Cognitive development in preterm infants: Birth to 8 years. *Developmental and Behavioral Pediatrics, 7*(2), 102-109.

Dawson, G., Frey, K., Panagiotides, H., Yamada, E., Hessel, D., & Osterling, J. (1999). Infants of depressed mothers exhibit atypical frontal electrical brain activity during interactions with mothers and with a familiar nondepressed adult. *Child Development, 70*, 1058-1066.

Diamond, A. (1985). Development of the ability to use recall to guide action, as indicated by infants' performance on A*B*. *Child Development, 56*, 868-883.

Diamond, A. (1993). Neuropsychological insights into the meaning of object concept development. In M. H. Johnson (Ed.), *Brain development and cognition: A reader* (pp. 208-247). Cambridge, MA: Blackwell.

Diamond, A., & Doar, B. (1989). The performance of human infants on a measure of frontal cortex function, the delayed response task. *Developmental Psychobiology, 22*(3), 271-294.

Diamond, A., & Goldman-Rakic, P. S. (1986). Comparative development of human infants and infant rhesus monkeys of cognitive functions that depend on the prefrontal cortex. *Neuropsychological Abstracts, 12*, 274.

Diamond, A., Kirkham, N., & Amso, D. (2002). Conditions under which young children can hold two rules in mind and inhibit a prepotent response. *Developmental Psychology, 38*(3), 352-362.

Diamond, A., & Lee, E. (2000). Inability of five-month-old infants to retrieve a contiguous object: A failure of conceptual understanding or of control of action? *Child Development, 71*(6), 1477-1494.

Diamond, A., Prevor, M. B., Callender, G., & Druin, D. P. (1997). Prefrontal cortex cognitive deficits in children treated early and continuously for PKU. *Monographs of the Society for Research in Child Development, 62*(4), 1-205.

Duffy, F. H., Als, H., & McAnulty, G. B. (1990). Behavioral and electrophysiological evidence for gestational age effects in healthy preterm and full-term infants studies two weeks after expected due date. *Child Development, 61*, 1271-1286.

Emsley, H. C., Wardle, S. P., Sims, D. G., Cheswick, M. L., & Souza, S. W. (1998). Increased survival and deteriorating developmental outcome in 23 to 25 week old gestation infants, 1990-1994 compared to 1984-1990. *Archives of Disease in Childhood, 78*, F99-F104.

Eslinger, P. J., Biddle, K., Pennington, B., & Page, R. B. (1999). Cognitive and behavioral development up to 4 years after early right frontal lobe lesion. *Developmental Neuropsychology, 15*(2), 157-191.

Eslinger, P. J., Grattan, L. M., Damasio, H., & Damasio, A. R. (1992). Developmental consequences of childhood frontal lobe damage. *Archives of Neurology, 49*, 764-769.

Eyal, F. G. (1993). The small-for-gestational-age preterm infant. In F. R. Witter & L. G. Keith (Eds.), *Textbook of prematurity: Antecedents, treatment, and outcome* (pp. 361-369). Boston, MA: Little, Brown.

Fletcher, J. M., Brookshire, B. L., Landry, S. H., Bohan, T. P., Davidson, K. C., Francis, D. J., et al. (1996). Attentional skills and executive functions in children with early hydrocephalus. *Developmental Neuropsychology, 12*(1), 53-76.

Fuster, J. M. (1991). Role of prefrontal cortex in delay tasks: Evidence from reversible lesion and unit recording in the monkey. In H. S. Levin & H. M. Eisenberg (Eds.), *Frontal function and dysfunction* (pp. 59-71). New York: Oxford University Press.

Fuster, J. M. (1997). *The prefrontal cortex: Anatomy, physiology, and neuropsychology of the frontal lobe*. New York: Lippincott-Raven.

Gathercole, S. E., & Pickering, S. J. (2000). Working memory deficits in children with low achievements in the national curriculum at 7 years of age. *British Journal of Educational Psychology, 70*, 177-194.

Gilles, F. H., Shankle, W., & Dooling, E. C. (1983). Myelinated tracts: Growth pattern. In F. H. Gilles, A. D. Leviton & E. C. Dooking (Eds.), *The developing human brain: Growth and epidemiologic neuropathology*. Baltimore: Williams & Wilkins.

Goldman-Rakic, P. S. (1994). Specification of higher cortical functions. In S. H. Broman & J. Grafman (Eds.), *Atypical cognitive deficits in developmental disorders: Implication for brain function* (pp. 3-17). Hillsdale, NJ: Lawrence Erlbaum.

Goldman-Rakic, P. S., & Rosvold, H. E. (1972). The effects of selective caudate lesions in infant and juvenile rhesus monkeys. *Brain Research, 42*, 53-66.

Grady, C. L. (1999). Neuroimaging and activation of the frontal lobes. In B. L. Miller & J. L. Cummings (Eds.), *The human frontal lobes: Functions and disorders* (pp. 196-230). New York: The Guilford Press.

Graham, S., & Harris, K. R. (1996). Addressing problems in attention, memory, and executive functioning. In G. R. Lyon & N. A. Krasnegor (Eds.), *Attention, memory, and executive function* (pp. 349-365). Baltimore: Paul H. Brookes.

Gregoire, M. C., Lefebvre, F., & Glorieux, J. (1998). Health and developmental outcomes at 18 months in very preterm infants with bronchopulmonary dysplasia. *Pediatrics, 101*(5), 856-860.

Guitton, D., Buchtel, H. A., & Douglas, R. M. (1985). Frontal lobe lesions in man cause difficulties in suppressing reflexive glances and in generating goal-directed saccades. *Experimental Brain Research, 58*, 455-472.

Hack, M., Friedman, H., & Fanaroff, A. A. (1996). Outcomes of extremely low birth weight infants. *Pediatrics, 98*(5), 931-937.

Harvey, J. M., O'Callaghan, M. J., & Mohay, H. (1999). Executive function of children with extremely low birthweight: A case control study. *Developmental Medicine and Child Neurology, 41*, 292-297.

Hecaen, H. (1964). Mental symptoms associated with tumors of the frontal lobe. In J. M. Warren & K. Akert (Eds.), *The frontal granular cortex and behavior*. New York: McGraw-Hill.

Hertzig, M. E. (1981). Neurological 'soft' signs in low-birthweight children. *Developmental Medicine and Child Neurology, 23*, 778-791.

Hofstadter, M., & Reznick, J. S. (1996). Response modality effects: Human infant delayed-response performance. *Child Development, 67*, 646-658.

Hoon, A., & Melhem, E. R. (2000). Neuroimaging: Applications in disorders of early brain development. *Developmental and Behavioral Pediatrics, 21*(4), 291-302.

Horobin, K., & Acredolo, L. (1986). The role of attentiveness, mobility history, and separation of hiding sites on Stage IV search behavior. *Journal of Experimental Child Psychology, 41*, 114-127.

Hunt, J. V., & Rhodes, L. (1977). Mental development of preterm infants during the first year. *Child Development, 48*, 204-210.

Huttenlocher, P. R. (1994). Synaptogenesis in human cerebral cortex. In G. Dawson & K. W. Fischer (Eds.), *Human behavior and the developing brain* (pp. 137-152). New York: The Guilford Press.

Jagust, W. (1999). Neuroimaging and the frontal lobes: Insight from the study of neurodegenerative diseases. In B. L. Miller & J. L. Cummings (Eds.), *The human frontal lobes: Functions and disorders* (pp. 107-122). New York: The Guilford Press.

Kaufer, D. I., & Lewis, D. A. (1999). Frontal lobe anatomy and cortical connectivity. In B. L. Miller & J. L. Cummings (Eds.), *The human frontal lobes: Functions and disorders* (pp. 27-44). New York: The Guilford Press.

Klebanov, P. K., Brooks-Gunn, J., & McCormick, M. C. (1994). Classroom behavior of very low birth weight elementary school children. *Pediatrics, 94*(5), 700-708.

Koller, H., Lawson, K., Rose, S. A., Wallace, I., & McCarton, C. (1997). Patterns of cognitive development in very low birth weight children during the first six years of life. *Pediatrics, 99*(3), 383-389.

Landry, S. H., Denson, S. E., & Swank, P. R. (1997). Effects of medical risk and socioeconomic status on the rate of change in cognitive and social development for low birth weight children. *Journal of Clinical and Experimental Neuropsychology, 19*(2), 261-274.

Laucht, M., Esser, G., & Schmidt, M. H. (1997). Developmental outcome of infants born with biological and psychosocial risks. *Journal of Child Psychology and Psychiatry and Allied Disciplines, 38*(7), 843-853.

Lepage, M., Beaudoin, G., Boulet, C., O'Brien, I., Marcantoni, W., Bourgouin, P., et al. (1999). Frontal cortex and the programming of repetitive tapping movements in man: Lesion effects and functional neuroimaging. *Cognitive Brain Research, 8*, 17-25.

Levin, H. S., Song, J., Ewing-Cobbs, L., & Roberson, G. (2001). Porteus Maze performance following traumatic brain injury in children. *Neuropsychology, 15*(4), 557-567.

Levine, S. C. (1993). Effects of early unilateral lesions: Changes over the course of development. In G. Turkewitz & D. A. Devenny (Eds.), *Developmental time and timing* (pp. 143-165). Hillsdale, NJ: Lawrence Erlbaum.

Lewinsohn, P. M., Zieler, R. E., Libet, J., Eyeberg, S., & Nielson, G. (1972). Short-term memory: A comparison between frontal and nonfrontal right- and left-hemisphere brain damaged patients. *Journal of Comparitive Physiology and Psychology, 81*, 248-255.

Luciana, M., Lindeke, L., Georgieff, M., Mills, M., & Nelson, C. A. (1999). Neurobehavioral evidence for working-memory deficits in school-aged children with histories of prematurity. *Developmental Medicine and Child Neurology, 41*, 521-533.

Marenco, S., Coppola, R., Daniel, D. G., Zigun, J. R., & Weinberger, D. R. (1993). Regional cerebral blood flow during the Wisconsin Card Sorting Test in normal subjects studied by xenon-133 dynamic SPECT: Comparison of absolute values, percent distribution values, and covariance analysis. *Psychiatry Research: Neuroimaging, 50*, 177-192.

Mateer, C. A., & Williams, D. (1991). Effects of frontal lobe injury in childhood. *Developmental Neuropsychology, 7*(2), 359-376.

McCall, R. B. (1994). What process mediates predictions of childhood IQ from infant habituation and recognition memory? Speculations on the roles of inhibition and rate of information processing. *Intelligence, 18*, 107-125.

McCarton, C. M., Wallace, I. F., Divon, M., & Vaughan, H. G. (1996). Cognitive and neurologic development of the premature, small for gestational age infant through age 6: Comparison by birth weight and gestational age. *Pediatrics, 98*(6), 1167-1178.

McDowell, S., Whyte, J., & D'Esposito, M. (1997). Working memory impairment in traumatic brain injury: Evidence from a dual-task paradigm. *Neuropsychologia, 35*(10), 1341-1353.

Milner, B. (1963). Effects of different brain lesions on card sorting. *Archives of Neurology, 9*, 90-100.

Milner, B. (1968). Disorders of memory after brain lesions in man. *Neuropsychologia, 6*, 175-179.

Molfese, V., & Thomson, B. (1985). Optimality versus complications: Assessing predictive values of perinatal scales. *Child Development, 56*, 810-823.

Mouradian, L. E., Als, H., & Coster, W. J. (2000). Neurobehavioral functioning of healthy preterm infants of varying gestational ages. *Developmental and Behavioral Pediatrics, 21*(6), 408-416.

Msall, M. E., Buck, G. M., Rogers, B. T., Mereke, D., Catanzaro, N. L., & Zorn, W. A. (1991). Risk factors for major neurodevelopmental impairments and need for special education resources in extremely premature infants. *Journal of Pediatrics, 119*, 606-614.

Nakawatase, T. Y. (1999). Frontal lobe tumors. In B. L. Miller & J. L. Cummings (Eds.), *The human frontal lobes: Functions and disorders* (pp. 436-445). New York: The Guilford Press.

Neville, H. E., & Chase, H. P. (1971). Undernutrition and cerebella development. *Experimental Neurology, 33*(3), 485-497.

O'Shea, T. M., Klinepeter, L., Goldstein, D. J., Jackson, B. W., & Dillard, R. G. (1997). Survival and developmental disability in infants with birth weights of 501 to 800 grams, born between 1979 and 1994. *Pediatrics, 100*(6), 982-986.

Petrides, M. (1985). Deficits on conditional associative-learning tasks after frontal- and temporal-lobe lesions in man. *Neuropsychologia, 23*, 601-614.

Petrides, M. (1994). Frontal lobe and working memory: Evidence from investigations of the effects of cortical excisions in nonhuman primates. In F. Boller, H. Spinnler & J. A. Hendler (Eds.), *Handbook of neuropsychology* (Vol. 9, pp. 59-82). Amsterdam: Elsevier Science.

Petrides, M. (1996). Learning impairments following excisions of the primate frontal cortex. In H. S. Levin, H. M. Eisenberg & A. L. Benton (Eds.), *Frontal lobe function and dysfunction* (pp. 256-272). New York: Oxford University Press.

Piaget, J. (1954). *The construction of reality in the child.* New York: Basic Books.

Piecuch, R. E., Leonard, C. H., Cooper, B., & Sehring, S. A. (1997). Outcome of extremely low birth weight infants (500 to 999 grams) over a 12-year period. *Pediatrics, 100*(4), 633-637.

Pine, T. R. L., Jackson, J. C., & Bennett, F. C. (1995). Outcome of infants weighing less than 800 grams at birth:15 years' experience. *Pediatrics, 96*, 479-483.

Piper, M. C., Kunos, I., Willis, D. M., & Mazer, B. (1985). Effect of gestational age on neurological functioning of the very low-birthweight infant at 40 weeks. *Developmental Medicine and Child Neurology, 27*, 596-605.

Rickards, A. L., Kelly, E. A., Doyle, L. W., & Callanan, C. (2001). Cognition, academic progress, behavior and self-concept at 14 years of very low birth weight children. *Developmental and Behavioral Pediatrics, 22*(1), 11-18.

Rieger, M., & Gauggel, S. (2002). Inhibition of ongoing responses in patients with traumatic brain injury. *Neuropsychologia, 40*, 76-85.

Roberts, E., Bornstein, M. H., Slater, A. M., & Barrett, J. (1999). Early cognitive development and parental education. *Infant and Child Development, 8*, 49-62.

Roberts, J. R. J., & Pennington, B. F. (1996). An interactive framework for examining prefrontal cognitive processes. *Developmental Neuropsychology, 12*(1), 105-126.

Ross, G., Lipper, E., & Auld, P. A. M. (1996). Cognitive abilities and early precursors of learning disabilities in very-low-birthweight children with normal intelligence and normal neurological status. *International Journal of Behavioral Development, 19*(3), 563-580.

Ross, G., Tesman, J., Auld, P. M., & Nass, R. (1992). Effects of subependymal and mild intraventricular lesions on visual attention and memory in premature infants. *Developmental Psychology, 28*(6), 1067-1074.

Rutter, M. (1992). *Developing minds: Challenge and continuity across the life span*. London, England: Penguin.

Sawaguchi, T., & Goldman-Rakic, P. S. (1994). The role of D1-dopamine receptor in working memory: Local injections of dopamine antagonists into the prefrontal cortex of rhesus monkeys performing an oculomotor delayed-response task. *Journal of Neurophysiology, 71*(2), 515-528.

Scheibel, R. S., & Levin, H. S. (1997). Frontal lobe dysfunction following closed head injury in children: Findings from neuropsychology and brain imaging. In N. A. Krasnegor, G. R. Lyon & P. S. Goldman-Rakic (Eds.), *Development of the prefrontal cortex: Evolution, neurobiology, and behavior* (pp. 241-263). Baltimore: Paul H. Brookes.

Shallice, T., & Burgess, P. W. (1991). Deficits in strategy application following frontal lobe damage in man. *Brain, 114*, 727-741.

Siegel, L. S. (1989). The development of working memory in normally achieving and subtypes of learning disabled children. *Child Development, 60*, 973-980.

Siegel, L. S. (1992). A multivariate model for the early detection of learning disabilities. In C. W. Greenbaum & J. G. Auerbath (Eds.), *Longitudinal studies of children at psychological risk: Cross-national perspectives* (pp. 99-132). Norwood , NJ: Ablex.

Smith, K. E., Landry, S. H., Swank, P. R., Baldwin, C. D., Denson, S. E., & Wildin, S. (1996). The relation of medical risk and maternal stimulation with preterm infants' development of cognitive, language and daily living skills. *Journal of Child Psychology and Psychiatry, 37*(7), 855-864.

Sostek, A. M. (1992). Prematurity as well as intraventricular hemorrhage influence developmental outcome at 5 years. In S. L. Friedman, M. D. Sigman & I. E. Sigel (Eds.), *The psychological development of low-birthweight children* (Vol. 6, pp. 259-274). Norwood, NJ: Ablex.

Stuss, D. T. (1991). Interference effects on memory functions in postleukotomy patients: An attentional perspective. In H. S. Levin, H. M. Eisenberg & A. L. Benton (Eds.), *Frontal lobe function and dysfunction* (pp. 157-172). New York: Oxford University Press.

Synnes, A. R., Ling, E. W. Y., Whitfield, M. F., Mackinnon, M., Lopes, L., Wang, G., et al. (1994). Perinatal outcomes of a large cohort of extremely low gestational age infants (twenty-three to twenty-eight completed weeks of gestation). *The Journal of Pediatrics, 125*(6), 952-960.

Taylor, H. G., Anselmo, M., Foreman, A. L., Schatschneider, C., & Angelopoulos, J. (2000). Utility of kindergarten teacher judgments in identifying early learning problems. *Journal of Learning Disabilities, 33*(2), 200-210.

Taylor, H. G., Hack, M., Klein, N., & Schatschneider, C. (1995). Achievement in children with birth weights less than 750 grams with normal cognitive abilities: Evidence for specific learning disabilities. *Journal of Pediatric Psychology, 20*(6), 703-719.

Taylor, H. G., Klein, N., Minich, N. M., & Hack, M. (2000). Middle-school-age outcomes in children with very low birthweight. *Child Development, 71*, 1495-1511.

Taylor, H. G., Klein, N., Schatschneider, C., & Hack, M. (1998). Predictors of early school age outcomes in very low birth weight children. *Developmental and Behavioral Pediatrics, 19*(4), 235-243.

Teuber, H.-L., & Rudel, R. G. (1962). Behavior after cerebral lesions in children and adults. *Developmental Medicine and Child Neurology, 4*, 3-20.

Thatcher, R. W. (1991). Maturation of the human frontal lobes: Physiological evidence for staging. *Developmental Neuropsychology, 7*(3), 397-419.

The Victorian Infant Collaborative Study Group. (1997). Outcome at 2 years of children 23-27 weeks' gestation born in Victoria in 1991-1992. *Journal of Pediatrics, 33*, 161-165.

Thompson, R. J., Gustafson, K. E., Oehler, J. M., Catlett, A. T., Brazy, J. E., & Coldstein, R. F. (1997). Developmental outcome of very low birth weight infants at four years of age as a function of biological risk and psychosocial risk. *Journal of Developmental and Behavioral Pediatrics, 18*(2), 91-96.

Ungerer, J. A., & Sigman, M. (1983). Developmental lags in preterm infants from one to three years of age. *Child Development, 54*, 1217-1228.

van de Bor, M., den Ouden, L., & Guit, G. L. (1992). Value of cranial ultrasound and magnetic resonance imaging in predicting neurodevelopmental outcome in preterm infants. *Pediatrics, 90*(2), 196-199.

Vasterling, J. J., Duke, L. M., Brailey, K., Constans, J. I., Allain, A. N., & Sutker, P. B. (2002). Attention, learning, and memory performances and intellectual resources in Vietnam veterans: PTSD and no disorder comparisons. *Neuropsychology, 16*(1), 5-14.

Welsh, M. C., & Pennington, B. F. (1988). Assessing frontal lobe functioning in children: View from developmental psychology. *Developmental Neuropsychology, 4*(3), 199-230.

Index

A

B

C

D

E

F

G

H

I

K

L

M

N

O

P

R

S

T

U

V

W

X